CANDIDA DIET COOKBOOK FOR VEGETARIANS

Easy-to-make and Delicious Plant-based recipes to healing your Gut, boosting your health and to Fight Candida Overgrowth

Dr. Mary D. Torres

TABLE OF CONTENT

INTRODUCTION

Candida overgrowth, a silent intruder within our bodies, has the potential to disrupt our lives in ways we might never have imagined. This seemingly harmless yeast, when allowed to flourish unchecked can wreak havoc on our health, causing a myriad of symptoms that affect both our physical and emotional well-being. The impact of Candida overgrowth on one's life can be profound, from relentless fatigue and digestive distress to skin issues, mood swings, and a weakened immune system. Yet, in the face of this challenge, there is hope.

As a professional dietitian with years of experience, I have witnessed firsthand the transformative effects of a well-structured Candida Diet for individuals seeking a vegetarian approach. It is a true testament to the remarkable resilience of the human body and the profound influence of dietary choices on our health.

This cookbook is a comprehensive guide crafted with the utmost care to assist you on your journey to better health and well-being. It is designed to not only help you understand the intricacies of Candida overgrowth but also to provide you with a treasure trove of mouthwatering recipes and nutritional to support your dietary transformation.

The journey may not always be easy, but with knowledge, dedication, and the right culinary tools, you can regain control over your health and reclaim your vitality.

CHAPTER 1: CANDIDA OVERGROWTH

What is Candida?

Candida is a type of yeast that is naturally found in small amounts in various parts of the human body, including the mouth, throat, intestines, and skin. It is considered a normal and harmless component of the body's microbiota which is the collection of microorganisms that reside in and on the body.

However, Candida can become problematic when it begins to overgrow or multiply in an uncontrolled manner. When this happens, it can lead to a condition known as Candida overgrowth or Candidiasis. Candida overgrowth most commonly affects the mucous membranes of the mouth and throat (oral thrush) or the genital area (vaginal yeast infections). Still, it can also impact other parts of the body, including the intestines and skin.

Causes of Candida Overgrowth

Candida overgrowth, also known as Candidiasis, can occur when there is an imbalance in the natural microbial communities that inhabit various parts of the body.

Several factors can contribute to this imbalance, allowing Candida yeast to overgrow but these are the common causes and contributing factors:

Antibiotic Use: Antibiotics are medications used to treat bacterial infections. While they are effective against harmful bacteria, they can also disrupt the balance of beneficial bacteria in the body, which normally help control Candida. This disruption can create an environment in which Candida can overgrow.

Weakened Immune System: A compromised immune system due to conditions like HIV/AIDS, autoimmune diseases, or ongoing stress can reduce the body's ability to keep Candida in check.

High Sugar Diet: Excessive consumption of sugary foods and refined carbohydrates can provide a ready source of energy for Candida yeast, promoting its growth. High Sugary diets can also lead to fluctuations in blood sugar levels, which may exacerbate Candida overgrowth.

Diabetes: People with uncontrolled diabetes are at an increased risk of Candida overgrowth because high blood sugar levels can promote the growth of yeast.

Hormonal Changes: Hormonal fluctuations, such as those that occur during pregnancy, menopause, or the use of birth control pills, can affect the body's pH levels and increase the risk of Candida overgrowth.

Weakened Digestive Function: Some conditions that affect digestion, such as irritable bowel syndrome (IBS) or digestive disorders, can disrupt the balance of microbes in the gut, potentially allowing Candida to thrive.

Excessive Alcohol Consumption: Too much alcohol intake can weaken the immune system and disrupt the balance of micro-organisms in the gut, this will make it easier for Candida to overgrow.

Use of Corticosteroids: The long-term use of corticosteroid medications, which are often prescribed for conditions like asthma, allergies, or autoimmune diseases can suppress the immune system and increase the risk of Candida overgrowth.

Chronic Stress: Prolonged stress can weaken the immune system and affect the body's ability to control Candida, making individuals more susceptible to overgrowth.

Tight or Non-Breathable Clothing: Excessive wearing of tight or non-breathable clothing, particularly in warm, moist environments, can create conditions conducive to the growth of Candida, especially in the genital area.

Symptoms and Health Implications

When Candida Overgrowth Occurs, It can manifest in a variety of symptoms that range from mild to severe. The symptoms of Candida overgrowth can affect different parts of the body and have a significant impact on an individual's overall health and well-being. However, these are some common symptoms and potential health implications associated with Candida overgrowth:

1. Oral Thrush:

Symptoms: White patches on the tongue, inner cheeks, or the roof of the mouth, along with discomfort or pain.

Health Implications: Oral thrush can interfere with eating and speaking comfortably. In severe cases, it may extend to the throat and esophagus, making swallowing painful.

2. Vaginal Yeast Infections:

Symptoms: Itching, burning, redness, and abnormal discharge in the genital area.

Health Implications: Recurrent vaginal yeast infections can be uncomfortable and distressing. They may also disrupt a person's intimate life and overall quality of life.

3. Digestive Issues:

Symptoms: Gas, bloating, diarrhea, or constipation, as well as abdominal discomfort.

Health Implications: Digestive problems can lead to nutritional deficiencies and affect the body's ability to absorb essential nutrients, potentially leading to fatigue and other health issues.

4. Fatigue and Weakness:

Symptoms: Persistent tiredness, lack of energy, and weakness.

Health Implications: Chronic fatigue can significantly impact one's daily life, productivity, and overall well-being.

5. Skin Problems:

Symptoms: Rashes, redness, itching, and skin irritation, particularly in warm, moist areas of the body.

Health Implications: Skin issues can be uncomfortable and affect self-esteem. Scratching can also lead to secondary infections.

6. Mood Swings and Mental Health Symptoms:

Symptoms: Mood swings, anxiety, depression, and cognitive difficulties.

Health Implications: Mental health symptoms can affect one's emotional well-being and cognitive function, impacting their quality of life and relationships.

7. Recurrent Infections:

Symptoms: Frequent yeast infections, urinary tract infections, or respiratory infections.

Health Implications: Recurrent infections can be a sign of weakened immunity and may require medical attention.

8. Immune System Weakness:

Symptoms: Frequent illnesses or slow recovery from illnesses.

Health Implications: A compromised immune system can make individuals more susceptible to other infections and health issues.

9. Allergies and Sensitivities:

Symptoms: New or increased allergies, sensitivities, or food intolerances.

Health Implications: Allergies and sensitivities can cause discomfort and may limit food choices, potentially affecting nutrition.

However, Candida overgrowth may not always be the main cause of these symptoms, as other underlying health conditions can produce similar effects.

Food to add Diet

When following the Candida Diet, it is important to focus on foods that help inhibit the growth of Candida yeast while providing essential nutrients to support your overall health. These are list of foods to include in your Candida Diet:

1. Non-Starchy Vegetables: These should form the foundation of your diet. They are rich in fiber, vitamins, and minerals while being low in sugars. Include a variety of vegetables like spinach, kale, broccoli, cauliflower, zucchini, bell peppers, and cucumbers.

2. Lean Proteins: Choose high-quality sources of protein, which include:

Plant-Based Proteins: Tofu, tempeh, legumes (such as lentils, chickpeas, and black beans), and quinoa.

3. Healthy Fats: Incorporate sources of healthy fats into your meals Such as:

Avocados: Rich in monounsaturated fats and fiber.

Nuts and Seeds: Almonds, walnuts, chia seeds, and flaxseeds provide healthy fats and fiber.

Olive Oil: Extra virgin olive oil is a good source of monounsaturated fats and antioxidants.

4. Low-Sugar Fruits: While fruits should be consumed in moderation due to their natural sugar content, you can include fruits that are lower in sugar such as:

Berries: Blueberries, strawberries, raspberries, and blackberries.

Green Apples: These are generally lower in sugar compared to other apple varieties.

Citrus Fruits: Lemons, limes, and grapefruits.

5. Probiotic Foods: Probiotics support a healthy gut environment. Incorporate foods like:

Yogurt: Choose plain, unsweetened yogurt with live cultures.

Kefir: A fermented milk drink with probiotics.

Sauerkraut: Fermented cabbage rich in beneficial bacteria.

Kimchi: A spicy fermented vegetable dish.

6. Whole Grains (in moderation): Some whole grains can be included in your diet, but keep portions small to moderate:

Quinoa: A complete protein source.

Millet: A gluten-free grain with a mild flavor.

Brown Rice: A whole grain option.

7. Antifungal Foods: Incorporate ingredients with natural antifungal properties into your cooking:

Garlic: Garlic has potent antifungal properties and can be added to many dishes.

Coconut Oil: Contains caprylic acid, which is known to inhibit Candida growth.

Herbs and Spices: Use oregano, thyme, and cinnamon, which have antifungal properties.

8. Fresh Herbs and Seasonings: You can enhance the flavor of your meals with fresh herbs like basil, cilantro, parsley, and seasonings like ginger and turmeric.

9. Beverages: Staying hydrated is crucial. Drink plenty of water, herbal teas, and, if desired, unsweetened almond or coconut milk.

Food to Stay Away From

If you want to follow the Candida Diet to manage Candida overgrowth, it's crucial to avoid certain foods that can promote the growth of Candida yeast or exacerbate your symptoms. Below are some of the foods you should avoid.

1. Sugars and Sweeteners:

Table Sugar: White sugar, brown sugar, and powdered sugar.

High-Fructose Corn Syrup: Found in many processed foods and sugary beverages.

Honey: A natural sweetener, but it's high in fructose.

Maple Syrup: Contains sugars that can feed Candida.

Agave Nectar: Despite its reputation as a healthier sweetener, it's high in fructose.

2. Refined Carbohydrates:

White Bread: Highly processed and quickly broken down into sugars.

White Rice: Lacks fiber and nutrients.

Pasta: Made from refined wheat flour, which can raise blood sugar levels.

Cereals: Many breakfast cereals are high in sugar and refined grains.

3. Alcohol:

Beer: Contains yeast and carbohydrates that can promote Candida growth.

Wine: Fermented with yeast and can contain residual sugars.

Spirits: While they don't contain sugars, alcohol can weaken the immune system.

4. Dairy Products (in some cases):

High-Lactose Dairy: Milk, ice cream, and some yogurts can be problematic for some individuals. Opt for lactose-free options if needed.

Soft Cheeses: Brie, Camembert, and blue cheese contain mold and may exacerbate Candida overgrowth.

5. Fruits High in Sugar:

Dried Fruits: Dates, raisins, and dried apricots are concentrated sources of sugar.

Tropical Fruits: Bananas, mangoes, and pineapples are higher in sugar.

6. Fruit Juices and Sweetened Beverages:

Fruit Juice: Even 100% fruit juice can be high in sugar.

Sodas and Sweetened Drinks: Loaded with sugars and artificial additives.

7. Processed and Convenience Foods:

Snack Bars: Many contain sugars, refined grains, and additives.

Fast Food: High in sugars, refined carbs, and unhealthy fats.

Packaged Snacks: Chips, crackers, and cookies often contain sugars and refined grains.

8. Condiments and Sauces:

Ketchup: Contains added sugars.

Mayonnaise: Some varieties have added sugars.

Soy Sauce: Typically contains wheat and is high in sodium.

9. Vinegar-Containing Foods:

Balsamic Vinegar: Contains sugars and can feed Candida.

Pickled Vegetables: Often pickled in vinegar.

10. Processed Meats:

Sausages: May contain sugars, preservatives, and fillers.

Bacon: Often cured with sugar.

11. Certain Grains:

Gluten-Containing Grains: Wheat, barley, and rye can be problematic for some individuals, especially if they have gluten sensitivity.

12. Moldy or Aged Cheeses:

Moldy Cheeses: Cheese varieties like gorgonzola, stilton, and Roquefort contain mold.

CHAPTER 2: VEGETARIANISM AND CANDIDA DIET

Why vegetarianism in candida diet?

A vegetarian Candida Diet is a dietary approach that combines the principles of the Candida Diet with the practice of vegetarianism. It involves eliminating foods that promote Candida overgrowth while adhering to a vegetarian lifestyle, which excludes meat and seafood but includes plant-based foods. These are some reasons why individuals may choose a vegetarian approach when following the Candida Diet:

Ethical and Environmental Reasons: Many people adopt a vegetarian lifestyle due to concerns about animal welfare and the environmental impact of meat production. Choosing a vegetarian Candida Diet allows them to align their dietary choices with these values.

Personal Preference: Some individuals simply prefer the taste and texture of plant-based foods over animal products. For them, a vegetarian Candida Diet offers a way to address Candida overgrowth while adhering to their dietary preferences.

Health Benefits of Plant-Based Diets: Vegetarian diets are often associated with various health benefits, including lower cholesterol levels, reduced risk of heart disease, and better weight management. Combining a Candida Diet with a vegetarian approach can offer a holistic approach to health and wellness.

Rich in Fiber and Nutrients: Plant-based diets are typically rich in fiber, vitamins, minerals, and antioxidants, which can support overall health and immune function. These nutrients are essential for managing Candida overgrowth and promoting healing.

Diversity of Plant-Based Foods: Vegetarian diets encourage the consumption of a wide variety of fruits, vegetables, legumes, nuts, and seeds. This diversity of foods can provide a range of nutrients and flavors, making the Candida Diet more enjoyable and sustainable.

Lower Saturated Fat Intake: Plant-based diets tend to be lower in saturated fats, which can be beneficial for heart health. Reducing saturated fat intake may also help with inflammation, which can be associated with Candida overgrowth.

Reduced Exposure to Antibiotics and Hormones: Animal products can sometimes contain residues of antibiotics and hormones used in animal farming. By avoiding meat and seafood, individuals may reduce their exposure to these substances, which can disrupt the balance of gut bacteria.

It's important to note that while a vegetarian Candida Diet can be effective in managing Candida overgrowth, it still requires careful attention to dietary choices. Vegetarians need to ensure they select foods that align with both the Candida Diet principles and their vegetarian lifestyle. This includes avoiding high-sugar plant-based foods and incorporating plenty of Candida-friendly vegetables, legumes, and plant-based proteins into their meals.

Benefit of Vegetarianism

Vegetarianism is a dietary lifestyle that excludes the consumption of meat, poultry, and seafood, and in some cases, animal by-products like gelatin and rennet. Many individuals choose vegetarianism for a variety of reasons, and it offers numerous potential benefits:

Improved Heart Health: Vegetarian diets are often associated with lower levels of saturated fat and cholesterol. This can lead to reduced risk factors for heart disease, such as high blood pressure and high cholesterol levels. Plant-based diets are also rich in heart-healthy nutrients like fiber, antioxidants, and potassium.

Weight Management: Vegetarian diets tend to be lower in calories and saturated fats compared to diets that include meat. As a result, vegetarians often find it easier to achieve and maintain a healthy weight. Plant-based diets can also be effective for weight loss and preventing obesity-related conditions.

Lower Risk of Chronic Diseases: Research has shown that vegetarian diets may be associated with a reduced risk of chronic diseases, including type 2 diabetes, certain types of cancer (such as colon, breast, and prostate cancer), and metabolic syndrome. The abundance of antioxidants and anti-inflammatory compounds in plant-based foods contributes to these benefits.

Better Digestive Health: Vegetarian diets are typically rich in dietary fiber, which promotes regular bowel movements and supports a healthy digestive system. This can help prevent constipation and reduce the risk of gastrointestinal disorders.

Improved Blood Sugar Control: Vegetarian diets can lead to better blood sugar control, making them suitable for individuals with diabetes or those at risk of developing the condition. The complex carbohydrates in plant-based foods help regulate blood glucose levels.

Lower Environmental Impact: Plant-based diets generally have a lower environmental footprint compared to diets heavy in animal products. Producing plant-based foods often requires fewer natural resources, produces fewer greenhouse gas emissions, and reduces deforestation and water pollution.

Ethical and Animal Welfare Concerns: Many vegetarians choose this lifestyle out of concern for animal welfare. They believe in reducing harm to animals by abstaining from consuming them or animal-derived products. This aligns with their ethical and moral values.

Cultural and Religious Beliefs: Some individuals follow vegetarian diets as part of their cultural or religious practices. For example, Hinduism, Buddhism, Jainism, and Seventh-day Adventism all have traditions that include vegetarianism as a central dietary component.

Improved Longevity: Research suggests that vegetarians may have a longer life expectancy and a reduced risk of premature death from lifestyle-related diseases.

Support for Sustainable Agriculture: Choosing plant-based diets promotes sustainable agriculture practices and reduces the demand for industrial livestock farming, which can have negative environmental and ethical consequences.

Important of Diet and Nutrition in Candida Overgrowth

Diet and nutrition play a pivotal role in managing Candida overgrowth. A well-planned diet can be a powerful tool in controlling Candida, alleviating symptoms, and supporting the body's natural ability to restore balance. Below are the key reasons why diet and nutrition are crucial in Candida overgrowth management:

Control of Candida Growth: Candida yeasts thrive on sugars and simple carbohydrates. By adopting a diet that restricts these sources of fuel, you can create an environment less conducive to Candida growth. This control is at the core of the Candida Diet.

Reduction of Symptoms: Candida overgrowth can lead to a wide range of symptoms, from digestive issues to skin problems and fatigue. Proper nutrition helps reduce the severity and frequency of these symptoms, improving your overall quality of life.

Support for Immune Function: A diet rich in essential nutrients, vitamins, and minerals is essential for a robust immune system. A well-functioning immune system can better control Candida and prevent its overgrowth.

Restoration of Gut Health: Candida overgrowth can disrupt the balance of beneficial and harmful microbes in the gut. A diet that supports a healthy gut microbiome is vital for long-term Candida control and overall well-being. Foods like yogurt, kefir, and fermented vegetables can help restore this balance.

Alleviation of Inflammation: Chronic inflammation is associated with Candida overgrowth. A diet high in anti-inflammatory foods, such as vegetables, fruits, and omega-3 fatty acids, can help reduce inflammation and promote healing.

Balanced Blood Sugar Levels: Fluctuations in blood sugar levels can exacerbate Candida overgrowth. A diet that focuses on complex carbohydrates, fiber, and balanced meals helps stabilize blood sugar levels, reducing the availability of sugar for yeast growth.

Promotion of Detoxification: Proper nutrition supports the body's natural detoxification processes, aiding in the elimination of toxins produced by Candida and supporting liver health.

Prevention of Nutrient Deficiencies: Candida overgrowth can interfere with nutrient absorption in the gut. A well-rounded diet ensures you receive essential nutrients, preventing deficiencies that could worsen Candida-related symptoms.

Improved Energy Levels: Managing Candida overgrowth can lead to increased energy levels and reduced fatigue, allowing you to engage in daily activities more effectively.

CHAPTER 3: Breakfast Delights

1. Avocado and Spinach Breakfast Bowl

Ingredients:

1 ripe avocado

1 cup fresh spinach leaves

2 tablespoons lemon juice

Salt and pepper to taste

Instructions:

Mash the avocado in a bowl.

Add lemon juice, salt, and pepper. Mix well.

Serve over a bed of fresh spinach.

Benefits: This breakfast is rich in healthy fats, fiber, and vitamins, supporting gut health and providing sustained energy.

2. Chia Seed Pudding

Ingredients:

2 tablespoons chia seeds

1 cup unsweetened almond milk

1/2 teaspoon pure vanilla extract

Stevia or erythritol for sweetness (optional)

Fresh berries for topping

Instructions:

Mix chia seeds, almond milk, vanilla, and sweetener (if desired) in a jar.

Stir well, seal, and refrigerate overnight.

Top with fresh berries before serving.

Benefits: Chia seeds are a good source of fiber and omega-3 fatty acids, promoting digestive health and reducing inflammation.

3. Greek Yogurt Parfait

Ingredients:

1 cup plain Greek yogurt (unsweetened)

1/4 cup fresh berries (e.g., blueberries, raspberries)

2 tablespoons chopped nuts (e.g., almonds, walnuts)

Cinnamon for flavor (optional)

Instructions:

In a glass, layer Greek yogurt, berries, and chopped nuts.

Sprinkle with cinnamon, if desired.

Benefits: Greek yogurt provides probiotics for gut health, while berries and nuts offer antioxidants and healthy fats.

4. Almond Flour Pancakes

Ingredients:

1 cup almond flour

2 eggs, 1/4 cup unsweetened almond milk

1/2 teaspoon baking powder, 1/2 teaspoon vanilla extract

Stevia or erythritol for sweetness (optional)

Coconut oil for cooking

Instructions:

In a bowl, mix almond flour, eggs, almond milk, baking powder, vanilla, and sweetener (if desired) until smooth.

Heat coconut oil in a pan over medium heat.

Pour pancake batter onto the pan and cook until bubbles form, then flip and cook until golden brown.

Benefits: These pancakes are grain-free and low in sugar, making them suitable for a Candida Diet.

5. Veggie Scramble

Ingredients:

2 eggs (or egg substitute for vegans)

Chopped vegetables (e.g., bell peppers, tomatoes, spinach)

Coconut oil for cooking

Herbs and spices for flavor (e.g., basil, oregano)

Salt and pepper to taste

Instructions:

Heat coconut oil in a pan over medium heat.

Add chopped vegetables and sauté until slightly softened.

Whisk eggs in a bowl and pour over the vegetables.

Cook until the eggs are set, stirring occasionally.

Season with herbs, spices, salt, and pepper.

Benefits: This protein-packed breakfast is rich in fiber and vitamins from the vegetables, supporting digestive health.

6. Coconut Yogurt with Berries

Ingredients:

Unsweetened coconut yogurt

Fresh mixed berries (e.g., strawberries, blackberries, raspberries)

Unsweetened shredded coconut for topping

Instructions:

Spoon coconut yogurt into a bowl.

Top with fresh mixed berries and shredded coconut.

Benefits: Coconut yogurt is dairy-free and low in sugar, and berries provide antioxidants and fiber.

7. Spinach and Mushroom Omelets

Ingredients:

2 eggs (or egg substitute for vegans)

Handful of fresh spinach leaves

Sliced mushrooms

Coconut oil for cooking

Salt and pepper to taste

Instructions:

Heat coconut oil in a pan over medium heat.

Add sliced mushrooms and sauté until they release moisture.

Add spinach leaves and sauté until wilted.

Whisk eggs in a bowl and pour over the vegetables.

Cook until the eggs are set, then fold the omelet in half.

Season with salt and pepper.

Benefits: This omelet is packed with protein, vitamins, and minerals from the spinach and mushrooms.

8. Almond Butter and Berry Wrap

Ingredients:

Almond butter (unsweetened)

Romaine lettuce leaves

Fresh berries (e.g., raspberries, blackberries)

Instructions:

Spread almond butter on romaine lettuce leaves.

Place fresh berries on top.

Roll up the leaves to create wraps.

Benefits: This quick and easy breakfast is rich in healthy fats, fiber, and antioxidants.

9. Green Smoothie

Ingredients:

Handful of spinach or kale

1/2 avocado

Unsweetened almond milk

Stevia or erythritol for sweetness (optional)

Ice cubes

Instructions:

Blend spinach or kale, avocado, almond milk, and sweetener (if desired) until smooth.

Add ice cubes and blend again until well combined.

Benefits: Green smoothies are nutrient-dense and support detoxification and digestive health.

10. Broccoli and Red Pepper Frittata

Ingredients:

4 eggs (or egg substitute for vegans)

Chopped broccoli florets

Chopped red bell pepper, Coconut oil for cooking

Salt and pepper to taste

Instructions:

Heat coconut oil in an oven-safe pan over medium heat.

Add chopped broccoli and red bell pepper and sauté until slightly softened.

Whisk eggs in a bowl and pour over the vegetables.

Cook until the edges are set, then transfer the pan to a preheated oven and broil until the top is golden brown.

Season with salt and pepper.

Benefits: This frittata is a protein-rich breakfast with the goodness of vegetables.

11. Vegan Chia Seed Breakfast Bowl

Ingredients:

2 tablespoons chia seeds

1 cup unsweetened almond milk

1/2 teaspoon pure vanilla extract

Stevia or erythritol for sweetness (optional)

Sliced almonds and berries for topping

Instructions:

Mix chia seeds, almond milk, vanilla, and sweetener (if desired) in a jar.

Stir well, seal, and refrigerate overnight.

Top with sliced almonds and berries before serving.

Benefits: This vegan chia seed bowl is a nutrient-packed breakfast option rich in fiber and healthy fats.

12. Cucumber and Avocado Smoothie

Ingredients:

1 cucumber

1/2 avocado

Unsweetened almond milk

Fresh mint leaves

Stevia or erythritol for sweetness (optional)

Ice cubes

Instructions:

Blend cucumber, avocado, almond milk, fresh mint leaves, and sweetener (if desired) until smooth.

Add ice cubes and blend again until well combined.

Benefits: This refreshing smoothie is hydrating and supports digestive health.

13. Vegan Tofu Scramble

Ingredients:

1/2 block of firm tofu, crumbled

Chopped vegetables (e.g., bell peppers, onions, spinach)

Turmeric and paprika for flavor

Nutritional yeast for a cheesy taste (optional)

Salt and pepper to taste

Instructions:

Sauté chopped vegetables in a pan until tender.

Add crumbled tofu and cook until heated through.

Season with turmeric, paprika, nutritional yeast (if desired), salt, and pepper.

Benefits: This vegan scramble is a protein-packed, savory breakfast option.

14. Quinoa Breakfast Bowl

Ingredients:

Cooked quinoa

Sliced bananas

Chopped nuts (e.g., almonds, walnuts)

Cinnamon for flavor

Unsweetened almond milk

Instructions:

Place cooked quinoa in a bowl.

Top with sliced bananas, chopped nuts, and a sprinkle of cinnamon.

Add almond milk to achieve your desired consistency.

Benefits: Quinoa is a high-protein grain that provides sustained energy throughout the morning.

15. Spinach and Mushroom Breakfast Wrap

Ingredients:

Whole-grain or gluten-free tortilla

Sautéed spinach and mushrooms

Sliced avocado

Salsa for flavor

Instructions:

Lay out a tortilla and add sautéed spinach and mushrooms.

Top with sliced avocado and salsa.

Roll up the tortilla to create a wrap.

Benefits: This savory breakfast wrap is packed with fiber, vitamins, and minerals from the vegetables.

Short Benefits Summary:

- These breakfast recipes are suitable for a Candida Diet for vegetarians and prioritize low-sugar, whole, and unprocessed ingredients.
- They provide essential nutrients, support gut health, and help manage Candida overgrowth.
- Many of these recipes are rich in fiber, healthy fats, and plant-based proteins, making them satisfying and nutritious options for your morning meal.

CHAPTER 4: Wholesome Lunches

1. Quinoa and Vegetable Stir-Fry

Ingredients:

Cooked quinoa

Mixed stir-fry vegetables (e.g., bell peppers, broccoli, carrots)

Tamari sauce (gluten-free soy sauce)

Garlic and ginger for flavor

Coconut oil for cooking

Instructions:

Heat coconut oil in a pan over medium heat.

Sauté garlic and ginger.

Add mixed vegetables and stir-fry until tender.

Add cooked quinoa and tamari sauce, tossing to combine.

Benefits: This quinoa stir-fry is a nutrient-packed meal rich in protein, fiber, and antioxidants from the vegetables.

2. Lentil and Vegetable Soup

Ingredients:

Green or brown lentils

Chopped mixed vegetables (e.g., onions, carrots, celery)

Vegetable broth (yeast-free)

Garlic and herbs for flavor

Olive oil for sautéing

Instructions:

Sauté chopped vegetables in olive oil until softened.

Add lentils and vegetable broth.

Simmer until lentils are tender.

Season with garlic and herbs.

Benefits: Lentils are a great source of plant-based protein and fiber, making this soup filling and nutritious.

3. Chickpea Salad

Ingredients:

Cooked chickpeas

Chopped cucumber, tomatoes, and red onion

Lemon juice and olive oil dressing

Fresh herbs (e.g., parsley, cilantro)

Salt and pepper to taste

Instructions:

Combine chickpeas, chopped vegetables, and herbs in a bowl.

Drizzle with lemon juice and olive oil dressing.

Season with salt and pepper.

Benefits: Chickpeas provide protein and fiber, while fresh vegetables and herbs add vitamins and minerals to this salad.

4. Cauliflower Rice and Vegetable Bowl

Ingredients:

Cauliflower rice (grated cauliflower)

Sautéed mixed vegetables (e.g., bell peppers, zucchini, broccoli)

Coconut aminos (soy-free alternative to soy sauce)

Garlic and ginger for flavor

Sesame seeds for garnish (optional)

Instructions:

Sauté garlic and ginger in a pan.

Add cauliflower rice and mixed vegetables.

Drizzle with coconut aminos and cook until heated through.

Garnish with sesame seeds, if desired.

Benefits: This low-carb, vegetable-packed bowl is a great way to enjoy the flavors of stir-fry without the traditional rice.

5. Spinach and Mushroom Salad with Avocado Dressing

Ingredients:

Fresh spinach leaves

Sliced mushrooms

Avocado, lemon, and garlic dressing

Chopped nuts (e.g., almonds, walnuts)

Salt and pepper to taste

Instructions:

Toss spinach leaves and sliced mushrooms in a bowl.

Drizzle with avocado, lemon, and garlic dressing.

Sprinkle chopped nuts on top and season with salt and pepper.

Benefits: This salad provides fiber, vitamins, healthy fats, and antioxidants from the spinach, mushrooms, and avocado.

6. Vegan Cauliflower and Broccoli Soup

Ingredients:

Chopped cauliflower and broccoli

Vegetable broth (yeast-free)

Onion and garlic for flavor

Coconut milk (unsweetened)

Turmeric and cumin for flavor

Olive oil for sautéing

Instructions:

Sauté onions and garlic in olive oil.

Add chopped cauliflower and broccoli.

Pour in vegetable broth and coconut milk.

Simmer until vegetables are tender.

Season with turmeric and cumin.

Benefits: This vegan soup is creamy and comforting, packed with cruciferous vegetables and anti-inflammatory spices.

7. Zucchini Noodles with Pesto

Ingredients:

Zucchini noodles (zoodles)

Homemade or store-bought pesto (without cheese)

Cherry tomatoes and pine nuts for topping

Fresh basil leaves for garnish

Instructions:

Toss zucchini noodles with pesto.

Top with cherry tomatoes, pine nuts, and fresh basil leaves.

Benefits: Zucchini noodles are a low-carb alternative to pasta, and pesto provides healthy fats and flavor.

8. Stuffed Bell Peppers

Ingredients:

Bell peppers (any color)

Quinoa or cauliflower rice

Sautéed vegetables (e.g., onions, tomatoes, spinach)

Tomato sauce (sugar-free)

Herbs and spices for flavor

Instructions:

Cut the tops off bell peppers and remove seeds.

Fill with a mixture of quinoa or cauliflower rice and sautéed vegetables.

Top with tomato sauce and herbs and spices.

Bake until peppers are tender.

Benefits: Stuffed bell peppers are a well-balanced meal with a variety of vegetables and a choice of quinoa or cauliflower rice.

9. Vegan Black Bean Soup

Ingredients:

Black beans (cooked or canned, unsalted)

Chopped onions, bell peppers, and tomatoes

Vegetable broth (yeast-free)

Cumin, chili powder, and paprika for flavor

Lime juice for garnish

Instructions:

Sauté onions, bell peppers, and tomatoes in a pot.

Add black beans and vegetable broth.

Season with cumin, chili powder, and paprika.

Simmer until flavors meld.

Serve with a squeeze of lime juice.

Benefits: This vegan black bean soup is rich in plant-based protein and fiber, with a hint of spice.

10. Spinach and Mushroom Stuffed Portobello Mushrooms

Ingredients:

Portobello mushroom caps

Sautéed spinach and mushrooms

Coconut oil for brushing, Herbs and spices for flavor

Nutritional yeast for a cheesy taste (optional)

Instructions:

Brush Portobello mushroom caps with coconut oil.

Stuff with sautéed spinach and mushrooms.

Season with herbs, spices, and nutritional yeast (if desired).

Bake until mushrooms are tender.

Benefits: Portobello mushrooms make a satisfying base for this savory, stuffed dish rich in vegetables.

11. Vegan Lentil Salad

Ingredients:

Cooked green or brown lentils

Chopped mixed vegetables (e.g., cucumbers, cherry tomatoes, red onion)

Fresh lemon and parsley dressing

Salt and pepper to taste

Instructions:

Combine cooked lentils and chopped vegetables in a bowl.

Drizzle with lemon and parsley dressing.

Season with salt and pepper.

Benefits: This vegan lentil salad is a protein-packed option with the fresh flavors of vegetables and lemon.

12. Vegan Cauliflower and Broccoli Rice Bowl

Ingredients:

Cauliflower rice and broccoli rice (grated)

Sautéed mixed vegetables (e.g., bell peppers, snow peas)

Coconut aminos (soy-free alternative to soy sauce)

Garlic and ginger for flavor

Chopped green onions for garnish

Instructions:

Sauté garlic and ginger in a pan.

Add cauliflower rice, broccoli rice, and mixed vegetables.

Drizzle with coconut aminos and cook until heated through.

Garnish with chopped green onions.

Benefits: This grain-free bowl is loaded with colorful vegetables and savory flavors.

13. Vegan Cabbage Rolls

Ingredients:

Cabbage leaves

Quinoa or cauliflower rice

Sautéed vegetable filling (e.g., onions, carrots, celery)

Tomato sauce (sugar-free)

Herbs and spices for flavor

Instructions:

Steam cabbage leaves until pliable.

Fill with a mixture of quinoa or cauliflower rice and sautéed vegetables.

Roll up the leaves and place in a baking dish.

Top with tomato sauce and season with herbs and spices.

Bake until cabbage is tender.

Benefits: Vegan cabbage rolls are a hearty, plant-based option with a variety of vegetables and a choice of quinoa or cauliflower rice.

14. Vegan Spinach and Artichoke Stuffed Mushrooms

Ingredients:

Large mushroom caps

Sautéed spinach and artichokes

Dairy-free cream cheese or cashew-based cheese

Garlic and herbs for flavor

Nutritional yeast for a cheesy taste (optional)

Instructions:

Fill mushroom caps with sautéed spinach and artichokes.

Top with dairy-free cream cheese or cashew-based cheese.

Season with garlic, herbs, and nutritional yeast (if desired).

Bake until mushrooms are tender.

Benefits: These stuffed mushrooms are a creamy and savory delight, featuring nutrient-rich spinach and artichokes.

15. Vegan Roasted Vegetable Bowl

Ingredients:

Roasted mixed vegetables (e.g., sweet potatoes, Brussels sprouts, carrots)

Quinoa or cauliflower rice, Tahini or lemon-tahini dressing

Fresh herbs for garnish (e.g., parsley, cilantro)

Instructions:

Roast mixed vegetables in the oven until tender.

Serve over a bed of quinoa or cauliflower rice.

Drizzle with tahini or lemon-tahini dressing.

Garnish with fresh herbs.

Benefits: This bowl is a colorful and flavorful way to enjoy a variety of roasted vegetables and grains.

Short Benefits Summary:

- These lunch recipes are suitable for a Candida Diet for vegetarians, focusing on whole, unprocessed ingredients.
- They offer a variety of vegetables, plant-based proteins, and flavors to keep your meals satisfying and nutritious.
- Many of these recipes are rich in fiber, vitamins, minerals, and antioxidants, promoting digestive health and overall well-being.

CHAPTER 5: Delectable Dinners

1. Baked Spaghetti Squash with Marinara Sauce

Ingredients:

Spaghetti squash

Sugar-free marinara sauce

Sautéed garlic and onions

Italian herbs and spices

Olive oil for drizzling

Instructions:

Cut the spaghetti squash in half lengthwise and remove seeds.

Drizzle with olive oil and season with garlic, onions, herbs, and spices.

Bake until tender and scrape the flesh into "spaghetti" strands.

Serve with marinara sauce.

Benefits: Spaghetti squash is a low-carb alternative to pasta, and the sauce is sugar-free, making this dish Candida-friendly.

2. Vegan Cauliflower Alfredo with Zoodles

Ingredients:

Zucchini noodles (zoodles)

Cauliflower Alfredo sauce (dairy-free)

Sautéed mushrooms and spinach

Garlic and nutritional yeast for flavor

Instructions:

Sauté mushrooms and spinach until tender.

Toss zucchini noodles with cauliflower Alfredo sauce.

Top with sautéed vegetables, garlic, and nutritional yeast.

Benefits: This vegan Alfredo dish is creamy and satisfying, with the added goodness of cauliflower and zoodles.

3. Vegan Lentil and Vegetable Curry

Ingredients:

Cooked brown or green lentils

Mixed sautéed vegetables (e.g., bell peppers, carrots, peas)

Vegan curry sauce (sugar-free)

Herbs and spices for flavor (e.g., turmeric, cumin)

Coconut oil for sautéing

Instructions:

Sauté mixed vegetables in coconut oil until tender.

Add cooked lentils and vegan curry sauce.

Season with herbs and spices.

Simmer until flavors meld.

Benefits: This vegan lentil curry is rich in plant-based protein, fiber, and aromatic spices.

4. Vegan Stuffed Bell Peppers

Ingredients:

Bell peppers (any color)

Quinoa or cauliflower rice

Sautéed vegetable filling (e.g., onions, tomatoes, spinach)

Vegan tomato sauce (sugar-free)

Herbs and spices for flavor

Instructions:

Cut the tops off bell peppers and remove seeds.

Fill with a mixture of quinoa or cauliflower rice and sautéed vegetables.

Top with vegan tomato sauce and season with herbs and spices.

Bake until peppers are tender.

Benefits: Vegan stuffed bell peppers are a well-rounded meal, featuring a variety of vegetables and a choice of quinoa or cauliflower rice.

5. Vegan Broccoli and Cashew Stir-Fry

Ingredients:

Sautéed broccoli florets

Cashew sauce (dairy-free)

Sautéed bell peppers and snap peas

Garlic and ginger for flavor

Coconut oil for sautéing

Instructions:

Sauté broccoli florets until tender.

Add sautéed bell peppers, snap peas, garlic, and ginger.

Drizzle with cashew sauce and toss to combine.

Benefits: This vegan stir-fry is rich in crunchy vegetables and creamy cashew sauce, without dairy or added sugars.

6. Vegan Eggplant Parmesan

Ingredients:

Sliced eggplant rounds

Vegan marinara sauce (sugar-free)

Vegan cheese (dairy-free)

Breadcrumbs (gluten-free)

Herbs and spices for flavor

Olive oil for baking

Instructions:

Dip eggplant slices in olive oil, then coat with breadcrumbs and spices.

Bake until golden brown.

Layer with marinara sauce and vegan cheese.

Bake until cheese is melted and bubbly.

Benefits: This vegan version of eggplant Parmesan is a satisfying, gluten-free option.

7. Vegan Thai Vegetable Curry

Ingredients:

Mixed sautéed vegetables (e.g., bell peppers, broccoli, carrots)

Vegan Thai curry sauce (sugar-free)

Fresh basil leaves for garnish

Coconut oil for sautéing

Instructions:

Sauté mixed vegetables in coconut oil until tender.

Add vegan Thai curry sauce and simmer until heated through.

Garnish with fresh basil leaves.

Benefits: This Thai vegetable curry is full of flavor, featuring a variety of colorful vegetables and aromatic herbs.

8. Vegan Cauliflower Rice and Vegetable Bowl

Ingredients:

Cauliflower rice (grated)

Sautéed mixed vegetables (e.g., bell peppers, zucchini, asparagus)

Vegan teriyaki sauce (sugar-free)

Sesame seeds for garnish (optional)

Instructions:

Sauté mixed vegetables until tender.

Add cauliflower rice and drizzle with vegan teriyaki sauce.

Cook until heated through.

Garnish with sesame seeds, if desired.

Benefits: This grain-free bowl is rich in vegetables and savory teriyaki flavor.

9. Vegan Spinach and Artichoke Stuffed Spaghetti Squash

Ingredients:

Spaghetti squash

Vegan spinach and artichoke dip (dairy-free)

Sautéed cherry tomatoes and spinach

Nutritional yeast for flavor (optional)

Olive oil for drizzling

Instructions:

Cut the spaghetti squash in half lengthwise and remove seeds.

Drizzle with olive oil and season with cherry tomatoes, spinach, and nutritional yeast.

Bake until tender and scrape the flesh into "spaghetti" strands.

Fill with vegan spinach and artichoke dip.

Benefits: This stuffed spaghetti squash is creamy and flavorful, without dairy or added sugars.

10. Vegan Cauliflower and Chickpea Curry

Ingredients:

Sautéed cauliflower florets and chickpeas

Vegan curry sauce (sugar-free)

Sautéed onions and garlic

Herbs and spices for flavor (e.g., coriander, cumin)

Coconut oil for sautéing

Instructions:

Sauté cauliflower florets and chickpeas in coconut oil until tender.

Add sautéed onions and garlic.

Drizzle with vegan curry sauce and season with herbs and spices.

Simmer until flavors meld.

Benefits: This vegan curry is a hearty and protein-rich option with the goodness of cauliflower and chickpeas.

11. Vegan Mediterranean Quinoa Bowl

Ingredients:

Cooked quinoa

Sautéed mixed vegetables (e.g., bell peppers, cherry tomatoes, cucumbers)

Vegan tzatziki sauce (dairy-free)

Kalamata olives for garnish

Fresh parsley for garnish

Instructions:

Combine cooked quinoa and sautéed vegetables in a bowl.

Drizzle with vegan tzatziki sauce.

Garnish with Kalamata olives and fresh parsley.

Benefits: This Mediterranean-inspired bowl is a refreshing and nutritious option with the flavors of the Mediterranean.

12. Vegan Cabbage and Mushroom Stew

Ingredients:

Sautéed cabbage and mushrooms

Vegetable broth (yeast-free)

Sautéed onions and garlic

Herbs and spices for flavor (e.g., thyme, rosemary)

Olive oil for sautéing

Instructions:

Sauté cabbage and mushrooms in olive oil until tender.

Add sautéed onions and garlic.

Pour in vegetable broth and season with herbs and spices.

Simmer until flavors meld.

Benefits: This vegan stew is a comforting and hearty option featuring cabbage and mushrooms.

13. Vegan Cauliflower Shepherd's Pie

Ingredients:

Mashed cauliflower topping

Vegan lentil and vegetable filling

Vegan gravy (sugar-free)

Herbs and spices for flavor

Instructions:

Prepare mashed cauliflower by steaming and mashing cauliflower florets.

Layer mashed cauliflower over vegan lentil and vegetable filling.

Drizzle with vegan gravy.

Season with herbs and spices.

Bake until golden brown.

Benefits: This vegan Shepherd's Pie is a wholesome and comforting dish with a cauliflower twist.

14. Vegan Ratatouille

Ingredients:

Sautéed ratatouille vegetables (e.g., eggplant, zucchini, bell peppers)

Vegan tomato sauce (sugar-free)

Herbs and spices for flavor (e.g., thyme, oregano)

Olive oil for sautéing

Instructions:

Sauté ratatouille vegetables in olive oil until tender.

Drizzle with vegan tomato sauce and season with herbs and spices.

Simmer until flavors meld.

Benefits: This vegan Ratatouille is a colorful and flavorful dish featuring an array of Mediterranean vegetables.

15. Vegan Thai Peanut Noodles

Ingredients:

Rice noodles (gluten-free)

Vegan peanut sauce (sugar-free)

Sautéed mixed vegetables (e.g., bell peppers, carrots, snow peas)

Crushed peanuts for garnish

Fresh cilantro for garnish

Instructions:

Cook rice noodles according to package instructions.

Toss with vegan peanut sauce and sautéed mixed vegetables.

Garnish with crushed peanuts and fresh cilantro.

Benefits: These vegan Thai peanut noodles are a tasty and satisfying dinner option with a rich peanut flavor.

Short Benefits Summary:

- These dinner recipes are suitable for a Candida Diet for vegetarians, focusing on whole, unprocessed ingredients.
- They provide a variety of vegetables, plant-based proteins, and flavors to keep your meals flavorful and Candida-friendly.
- Many of these recipes are rich in fiber, vitamins, minerals, and antioxidants, supporting digestive health and overall well-being.

CHAPTER 6: DESSERT

1. Berry Chia Pudding

Ingredients:

2 tablespoons chia seeds

1 cup unsweetened almond milk

Mixed berries (e.g., strawberries, blueberries)

Stevia or erythritol for sweetness (optional)

Instructions:

Mix chia seeds and almond milk in a jar.

Stir well, seal, and refrigerate overnight.

Top with mixed berries and sweetener before serving.

Benefits: This dessert is rich in fiber, antioxidants, and omega-3 fatty acids, supporting gut health and reducing inflammation.

2. Vegan Coconut Bliss Balls

Ingredients:

Shredded unsweetened coconut

Almond flour

Coconut oil (melted)

Stevia or erythritol for sweetness (optional)

Vanilla extract for flavor

Instructions:

Mix shredded coconut, almond flour, melted coconut oil, sweetener (if desired), and vanilla extract in a bowl.

Roll into bite-sized balls and refrigerate until firm.

Benefits: These vegan coconut bliss balls are a satisfying, no-bake dessert with healthy fats and natural sweetness.

3. Vegan Avocado Chocolate Mousse

Ingredients:

Ripe avocado

Unsweetened cocoa powder

Stevia or erythritol for sweetness (optional)

Vanilla extract for flavor

Instructions:

Blend ripe avocado, cocoa powder, sweetener (if desired), and vanilla extract until smooth.

Refrigerate until chilled.

Serve with a sprinkle of cocoa powder.

Benefits: This vegan chocolate mousse is creamy and rich, providing healthy fats and antioxidants.

4. Baked Cinnamon Apple Slices

Ingredients:

Apple slices

Cinnamon for flavor

Stevia or erythritol for sweetness (optional)

Lemon juice for freshness

Instructions:

Arrange apple slices in a baking dish.

Sprinkle with cinnamon, sweetener (if desired), and lemon juice.

Bake until tender.

Benefits: These baked cinnamon apple slices are a warm and comforting dessert without added sugars.

5. Vegan Almond Butter Cookies

Ingredients:

Almond butter (unsweetened)

Almond flour

Stevia or erythritol for sweetness (optional)

Vanilla extract for flavor

Instructions:

Mix almond butter, almond flour, sweetener (if desired), and vanilla extract in a bowl.

Form into cookie shapes on a baking sheet.

Bake until lightly golden.

Benefits: These vegan almond butter cookies are gluten-free and sugar-free, offering protein and healthy fats.

6. Vegan Chocolate Zucchini Brownies

Ingredients:

Grated zucchini

Unsweetened cocoa powder

Almond flour

Stevia or erythritol for sweetness (optional)

Vanilla extract for flavor

Instructions:

Mix grated zucchini, cocoa powder, almond flour, sweetener (if desired), and vanilla extract in a bowl.

Pour into a baking dish and bake until set.

Benefits: These vegan chocolate zucchini brownies are a sneaky way to include veggies in your dessert and are gluten-free.

7. Vegan Berry Sorbet

Ingredients:

Mixed berries (e.g., strawberries, raspberries)

Lemon juice for freshness

Stevia or erythritol for sweetness (optional)

Instructions:

Blend mixed berries and lemon juice until smooth.

Add sweetener (if desired) and blend again.

Freeze until it reaches a sorbet-like consistency.

Benefits: This vegan berry sorbet is a refreshing and naturally sweet dessert.

8. Vegan Carrot Cake Bites

Ingredients:

Grated carrots

Almond flour

Cinnamon and nutmeg for flavor

Stevia or erythritol for sweetness (optional)

Instructions:

Mix grated carrots, almond flour, cinnamon, nutmeg, and sweetener (if desired) in a bowl.

Roll into bite-sized balls and refrigerate until firm.

Benefits: These vegan carrot cake bites are a healthy and bite-sized dessert option.

9. Vegan Pumpkin Spice Muffins

Ingredients:

Pumpkin puree (unsweetened)

Almond flour

Pumpkin spice seasoning

Stevia or erythritol for sweetness (optional)

Vanilla extract for flavor

Instructions:

Mix pumpkin puree, almond flour, pumpkin spice, sweetener (if desired), and vanilla extract in a bowl.

Pour into muffin cups and bake until set.

Benefits: These vegan pumpkin spice muffins are a flavorful dessert without added sugars.

10. Vegan Lemon Poppy Seed Cake

Ingredients:

Almond flour

Lemon zest and juice for flavor

Poppy seeds

Stevia or erythritol for sweetness (optional)

Instructions:

Mix almond flour, lemon zest, lemon juice, poppy seeds, and sweetener (if desired) in a bowl.

Bake in a cake pan until golden.

Benefits: This vegan lemon poppy seed cake is a zesty and gluten-free dessert option.

11. Vegan Chocolate Dipped Strawberries

Ingredients:

Fresh strawberries

Dark chocolate (sugar-free)

Stevia or erythritol for sweetness (optional)

Instructions:

Melt dark chocolate and sweetener (if desired) in a microwave-safe bowl.

Dip fresh strawberries into the melted chocolate.

Place on parchment paper and refrigerate until set.

Benefits: These vegan chocolate-dipped strawberries are a delightful, antioxidant-rich treat.

12. Vegan Blueberry Coconut Popsicles

Ingredients:

Fresh blueberries

Unsweetened coconut milk

Stevia or erythritol for sweetness (optional)

Instructions:

Blend fresh blueberries, coconut milk, and sweetener (if desired) until smooth.

Pour into popsicle molds and freeze until solid.

Benefits: These vegan blueberry coconut popsicles are a cool and dairy-free dessert.

13. Vegan Cinnamon Raisin Rice Pudding

Ingredients:

Cooked brown rice

Almond milk (unsweetened)

Cinnamon and raisins for flavor

Stevia or erythritol for sweetness (optional)

Instructions:

Mix cooked brown rice, almond milk, cinnamon, raisins, and sweetener (if desired) in a pot.

Simmer until the mixture thickens.

Serve warm or chilled.

Benefits: This vegan rice pudding is a comforting dessert with a hint of cinnamon and natural sweetness.

14. Vegan Mixed Berry Parfait

Ingredients:

Mixed berries (e.g., strawberries, blueberries)

Vegan coconut yogurt (unsweetened)

Stevia or erythritol for sweetness (optional)

Chopped nuts (e.g., almonds, walnuts)

Instructions:

Layer mixed berries and vegan coconut yogurt in a glass.

Add sweetener (if desired) and chopped nuts for crunch.

Benefits: This vegan mixed berry parfait is a balanced dessert with a mix of fruits, yogurt, and nuts.

15. Vegan Chocolate Avocado Popsicles

Ingredients:

Ripe avocado

Unsweetened cocoa powder

Almond milk (unsweetened)

Stevia or erythritol for sweetness (optional)

Instructions:

Blend ripe avocado, cocoa powder, almond milk, and sweetener (if desired) until smooth.

Pour into popsicle molds and freeze until solid.

Benefits: These vegan chocolate avocado popsicles are creamy and chocolatey, without dairy or added sugars.

Short Benefits Summary:

- These dessert recipes are suitable for a Candida Diet for vegetarians, focusing on natural sweetness and low-glycemic ingredients.
- They offer a variety of flavors, textures, and nutrients while keeping sugar content in check.
- Many of these recipes feature antioxidant-rich fruits and healthy fats for a satisfying sweet treat.

CONCLUSION

This Candida Diet Cookbook for Vegetarians offers a diverse range of recipes that align with the principles of a Candida-friendly diet. By following these guidelines and adopting a vegetarian lifestyle, individuals dealing with Candida overgrowth can experience a multitude of benefits.

The cookbook provides a wealth of delicious and nutritious options, ranging from breakfast delights to satisfying dinners and guilt-free desserts. These recipes are tailored to the needs of those with Candida overgrowth, emphasizing whole, unprocessed ingredients and avoiding foods that can exacerbate the condition.

The benefits of this cookbook and a vegetarian lifestyle for Candida sufferers are numerous:

Balanced Nutrition: The recipes are thoughtfully crafted to provide balanced nutrition, ensuring that essential vitamins, minerals, and macronutrients are included to support overall health.

Digestive Health: By avoiding sugars, refined grains, and processed foods, this cookbook promotes a healthy gut environment, reducing the risk of Candida overgrowth and digestive discomfort.

Inflammation Reduction: Many of the ingredients used in these recipes have anti-inflammatory properties, which can help alleviate symptoms associated with Candida overgrowth.

Blood Sugar Management: The focus on low-glycemic ingredients helps stabilize blood sugar levels, preventing the spikes and crashes that can worsen Candida symptoms.

Plant-Based Proteins: Vegetarianism offers plant-based protein sources that are gentle on the digestive system and can help repair tissue damage caused by Candida.

Rich in Fiber: The recipes incorporate fiber-rich ingredients, promoting healthy digestion and regular bowel movements.

Antioxidant-Rich: Fruits and vegetables included in the recipes are packed with antioxidants, supporting the body's defense against oxidative stress.

WEEKLY MEAL PLANNER

Meal Planner

Date:

Monday	Tuesday	Wednesday
BREAKFAST LUNCH DINNER DESSERTS	BREAKFAST LUNCH DINNER DESSERTS	BREAKFAST LUNCH DINNER DESSERTS

Thursday	Friday	Saturday
BREAKFAST LUNCH DINNER DESSERTS	BREAKFAST LUNCH DINNER DESSERTS	BREAKFAST LUNCH DINNER DESSERTS

Sunday	
BREAKFAST LUNCH DINNER DESSERTS	NOTES:

Meal Planner

Date:

Monday	Tuesday	Wednesday
BREAKFAST	BREAKFAST	BREAKFAST
LUNCH	LUNCH	LUNCH
DINNER	DINNER	DINNER
DESSERTS	DESSERTS	DESSERTS

Thursday	Friday	Saturday
BREAKFAST	BREAKFAST	BREAKFAST
LUNCH	LUNCH	LUNCH
DINNER	DINNER	DINNER
DESSERTS	DESSERTS	DESSERTS

Sunday	
BREAKFAST	NOTES:
LUNCH	
DINNER	
DESSERTS	

Meal Planner

Date:

Monday	Tuesday	Wednesday
BREAKFAST	BREAKFAST	BREAKFAST
LUNCH	LUNCH	LUNCH
DINNER	DINNER	DINNER
DESSERTS	DESSERTS	DESSERTS

Thursday	Friday	Saturday
BREAKFAST	BREAKFAST	BREAKFAST
LUNCH	LUNCH	LUNCH
DINNER	DINNER	DINNER
DESSERTS	DESSERTS	DESSERTS

Sunday	
BREAKFAST	NOTES:
LUNCH	
DINNER	
DESSERTS	

Meal Planner

Date:

Monday	Tuesday	Wednesday
BREAKFAST	BREAKFAST	BREAKFAST
LUNCH	LUNCH	LUNCH
DINNER	DINNER	DINNER
DESSERTS	DESSERTS	DESSERTS

Thursday	Friday	Saturday
BREAKFAST	BREAKFAST	BREAKFAST
LUNCH	LUNCH	LUNCH
DINNER	DINNER	DINNER
DESSERTS	DESSERTS	DESSERTS

Sunday	NOTES:
BREAKFAST	
LUNCH	
DINNER	
DESSERTS	

Printed in Great Britain
by Amazon

54039633R00046